T0190861

Everyday Herbal Teamaking

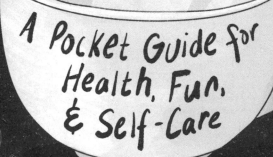

A Pocket Guide for Health, Fun, & Self-Care

GLENNA A. McLEAN

Microcosm Publishing

Portland, OR • Cleveland, OH

EVERYDAY HERBAL TEAMAKING
A pocket guide for health, fun, and self-care

© Glenna A. McLean, 2023

ISBN 9781648412028
This is Microcosm #733
First Published March, 2023
Cover by Lindsey Cleworth
Edited by Sarah Koch

This edition © Microcosm Publishing, 2023

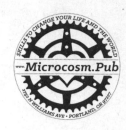

For a catalog, write or visit:
Microcosm Publishing
2752 N Williams Ave.
Portland, OR 97227
www.Microcosm.Pub/Tea

To join the ranks of high-class stores that feature Microcosm titles, talk to your local rep: In the U.S. **COMO** (Atlantic), **ABRAHAM** (Midwest), **BOB BARNETT** (Texas/Louisiana/Oklahoma), **IMPRINT** (Pacific), **TURNAROUND** (Europe), **UTP/MANDA** (Canada), **NEW SOUTH** (Australia/New Zealand), **GPS** in Asia, Africa, India, South America, and other countries, or **FAIRE** in the gift trade.

Did you know that you can buy our books directly from us at sliding scale rates? Support a small, independent publisher and pay less than Amazon's price at **www.Microcosm.Pub**

Library of Congress Cataloging-in-Publication Data
Names: McLean, Glenna A., 1945- author.
Title: Everyday herbal teamaking : a pocket guide for health, fun, and self-care / by Glenna A. McLean.
Description: [Portland] : Microcosm Publishing, 2023. | Summary: "This unfussy, spirited guide to 35 readily accessible herbs offers botanical names, medical reputations from various modern and historical sources, good-humoredly honest tasting notes, and illustrations to help identify what you've just foraged, grown, or bought at the herb shop or health food store. With teacher and tea aficionado Glenna McLean as your guide, travel back in time by enjoying a blend of herbs that King Tut savored, a tea that was thought to ward off the Plague in the 14th Century, and the herbs imbibed by druids at Stonehenge and Puritan church services. Quaff brews purported to bring you courage, quench (or ignite) lust, ward off scurvy, and soothe stress and pain. Includes warnings and contraindications so you can pursue your herbal tea habit safely and happily for years to come"-- Provided by publisher.
Identifiers: LCCN 2022050559 | ISBN 9781648412028 (trade paperback)
Subjects: LCSH: Herbal teas. | Herbs. | LCGFT: Cookbooks.
Classification: LCC TX415 .M39 2023 | DDC 641.3/372--dc23/eng/20221108
LC record available at https://lccn.loc.gov/2022050559

MICROCOSM · PUBLISHING

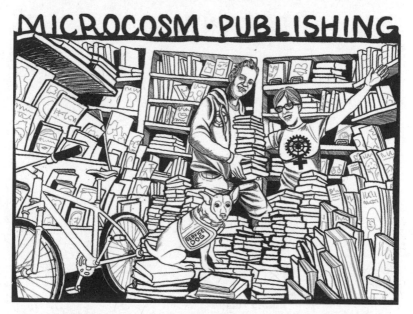

MICROCOSM PUBLISHING is Portland's most diversified publishing house and distributor with a focus on the colorful, authentic, and empowering. Our books and zines have put your power in your hands since 1996, equipping readers to make positive changes in their lives and in the world around them. Microcosm emphasizes skill-building, showing hidden histories, and fostering creativity through challenging conventional publishing wisdom with books and bookettes about DIY skills, food, bicycling, gender, self-care, and social justice. What was once a distro and record label started by Joe Biel in a drafty bedroom was determined to be *Publisher's Weekly's* fastest growing publisher of 2022 and has become among the oldest independent publishing houses in Portland, OR and Cleveland, OH. We are a politically moderate, centrist publisher in a world that has inched to the right for the past 80 years.

Global labor conditions are bad, and our roots in industrial Cleveland in the 70s and 80s made us appreciate the need to treat workers right. Therefore, our books are MADE IN THE USA

CONTENTS

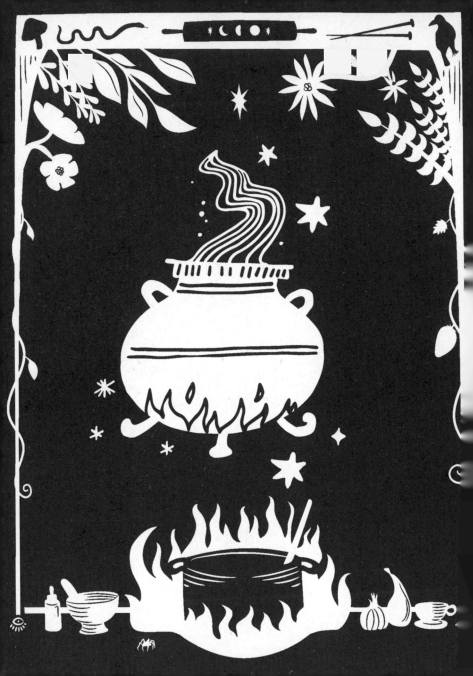

Introduction

When I went on my last health food kick, I became enthralled by the myriad of herbal teas out there. They all seem to have this magical, mystical aura about them. My Aquarian side urged me to throw caution to the winds, buy one of everything, and generally run amok.

But I also have a strong streak of Scots-Capricorn running through my veins. There was this small voice that warned me to hold onto my money and find out what I was about to put into my body. What in heaven's name would it do for me or to me and what in the hell would it taste like?

I searched for some sort of uncomplicated guide to tell me what I wanted to know. Since I couldn't find it, I decided to write one myself.

This book is meant to be fun. It is not a medical compendium nor is it meant to be used for prescriptions. It's just a general guide to tuck into your jeans or download on your phone and take along with you when you set out to sample herbal teas.

These teas can be found almost anywhere nowadays: a natural foods store, vitamin stores, grocery stores, your local drug store, etc. If you are a naturalist and know what you're doing, you can find tea fixin's growing in your yard, in the forest, down the block, or, in my case, growing under the sink, if it comes to that.

Why Drink Herbal Tea?

There are lots of reasons for buying and drinking herbal teas, not the least of which is money. With coffee prices rising steadily and more and more research making claims of caffeine-linked ailments, it's time to start taking self-sufficient, self-sustaining living and drinking styles seriously.

Herbal teas also have time-traveling properties to them: one sip and you can be transported back to almost any point in time. There is a tea used to deal with the Black Plague. Some were drunk by King Tut. One or two appeared at Druid ceremonies at Stonehenge. Even during the interminable Puritan church services, herbs were used.

Most herbal teas contain a wealth of various vitamins, minerals, chemicals, and trace elements that your body needs and can use in a (mostly) palatable form, and new science about these herbs is coming out every day. Happily, many of these teas are downright delicious and make more than acceptable replacements for your Lipton's, Tetley, Red Rose, whatever. In the interests of fair disclosure, there are also some herbal teas that, while they may be good for you, taste-wise they would give street rats the dry heaves. These will be duly noted.

The most important point is that drinking herbal tea can be fun. "Fun!?" you ask. "Tea is fun? Can anyone have a life that is that dull?" Well, yes—mine is—but that's another book.

Presentation

I have reviewed thirty-five of the most popular herbal teas. These reviews are divided into six categories: botanical names, parts used, their medicinal reputations, tasters' evaluations, a report card grade, and their their traditional and modern lore.

By fair means and foul (photographs from faculty Christmas parties, bribery, out and out threats of physical force), I was able to persuade many fellow teachers to agree to volunteer to sample the teas and fill in a brief reaction paper about them. Therefore, the assessments are purely subjective, as are the grades. The grading system is simple: A++ is the best; Z is the pits.

The botanical names are included because there are many herbs that look very similar, share the same name, or have various local names. The specific parts used for brewing are mentioned in case you wish to grow or gather your own. While most herbs are perfectly safe, occasionally some can present a problem if the wrong plant parts are used. Before you freak out, remember that while rhubarb stems are delicious in a pie, rhubarb leaves will make you a sick, sick (and possibly dead) puppy if you eat them. That's why you never see rhubarb in grocery stores with the leaves still on them. And, by the way, the same goes for potatoes. While the tubers are big yummy, the leaves are deadly. Feel better now?

FYI: One of the herbs that scared the living daylights out of me was black cohosh. It was very fashionable for a while, with all kinds of wonderful claims about its properties. My sister (and many others) used it, but she stopped when she began feeling unwell. She had medical tests done and tested positive for liver cancer. Luckily, she had a doctor who was brilliant and asked her if she was taking black cohosh. After a month of not drinking the cohosh, her liver was retested and she came up clean. Apparently, her case was not unusual.

I have tried to point out other possible troublemakers in this book but, on the whole, it's probably better to stick to the commercially sold herbs and plants—unless you really are a plant expert. In the same vein, those who are pregnant should always speak with their doctor before introducing anything new into their system; many of these herbs can have detrimental effects during pregnancy.

I have also included some of the most commonly mentioned medicinal properties ascribed to these teas through the centuries. Herbal teas are not a replacement for medicine, nor does this book intend that you use them as such. However, their traditional uses and the lore surrounding their benefits are frequently being corroborated by modern medical research.

Helpful Hints

When using bagged teas, try using two bags at a time per cup for more body and flavor. There never seemed to be enough real flavor when using just one bag. However, when using the loose pack teas, start with only one-half teaspoon per cup. For some reason, the loose teas seem more potent.

Allow the bags to steep for four or five minutes. (I know this could get me kicked out of the tea lovers' club, but I nuke the tea for a full five minutes. But that's just me.) From there you can drink it straight or add whatever flavor enhancers you enjoy: milk, honey, lemon, chopped broccoli—whatever.

Gratitude

I would indeed be remiss were I not to express my gratitude to the long-suffering faculty of Robert Moses Junior High in North Babylon, New York. These poor devils put up with me and (mostly) willingly (mostly) drank down gallons of some of the strangest stuff they had ever tried. Even our principal, Carl Smith, consented to be dragged into the act.

I should also mention my adorable students who annoy, nag, threaten, bully, and protect me: Richie, Jim, Christopher, Pete, Joe, Deb, Anthony, Gail, Doug, David, Melanie, and Ed.

Teacher still loves you all!

I would be remiss in not thanking the tireless (and always correct) Sarah Koch for the editing she did to bring order out of chaos. You're amazing.

Most important are Michael and Brian who kept after me until I finished this project—which ultimately became part of my Master's thesis. I have been very lucky to have you all in my life.

This book is especially dedicated to the memory of my Michael. The best thing that ever happened to me.

1. ANGELICA

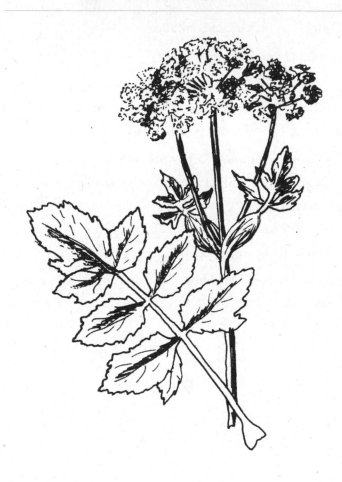

BOTANICAL NAME	*Angelica arcangelica*
PARTS USED	Leaves, stems, roots
MEDICINAL REPUTATION	Allegedly, about all it doesn't do is cure politicians of lying.
	Calms nervous or upset stomach.
	Promotes urination and perspiration.
	Speeds healing of wounds.
	Relaxes muscle spasms.
	"Cures" hydrophobia, asthma, and snakebite.
	Cools lust.
	Eases pain of gout and toothache.
	A specific cure for the Black Plague.
REACTION	Whew! Very strong spicy/musky taste; like root beer on steroids.
GRADE	B+

TRADITIONAL AND MODERN LORE

Angelica was delivered to a monk in a medieval monastery by the Archangel Michael during the Middle Ages. The monk dreamed he had a conversation with Michael. In the dream, the monk was instructed how to prepare the plant to cure those who had contracted the Plague. Ever since, the plant is said to bloom on St. Michael's Day. This could be tricky since there are several St. Michael's Days depending on where in the Christian world you live.

Perhaps uncoincidentally, its juice was also used to ward off evil spirits and/or witches who avoided the plant like the plague.

While there is limited proven research on Angelica's health benefits, there are some intriguing experiments. One is in breast cancer research, but it is still in the early stages of rat and *in vitro* trials. Some of the traditional attributes for improving appetite loss and relieving tummy upset and gas have been substantiated and approved by the German FDA (Commission E). Research is also looking into angelica's value in relieving arthritis pain and its possible anti-inflammatory properties, and The World Journal of Gastroenterology has suggested researching angelica's role in relieving Irritable bowel Syndrome (IBS).

It may increase sensitivity to sunlight—but as usual—this is a problem only when angelica tea is taken in large amounts.

CAUTION: Do not use if pregnant. Actually, don't use a lot of anything new and/or unusual during pregnancy.

2. ANISE

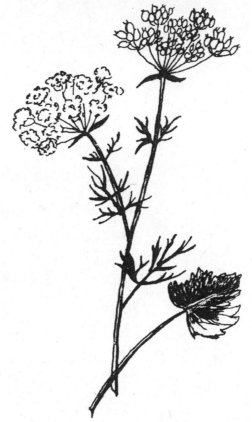

BOTANICAL NAME	*Pimpinella anisum*
PARTS USED	Seeds and leaves

MEDICINAL REPUTATION	Sweetens breath.
	Stimulates the appetite.
	An antispasmodic and antiflatulent.
	Once used to treat young epileptics.
REACTION	Licorice-y with a hint of celery; kind of pleasant.
GRADE	B+

TRADITIONAL AND MODERN LORE

The ancient Egyptians used anise as a preservative for mummy innards. And, according to various papyri describing the medical practices of the Egyptians, anise seeds and oil were often used for serious tummy ailments as well—nausea, gas, diarrhea.

More modern research has indicated that anise oil capsules, taken over month-long protocols, seem to reduce the symptoms of Irritable Bowel Syndrome. ". . . Aniseed essential oil improved symptoms of IBS including abdominal discomfort and pain, bloating, diarrhea, constipation, and gastroesophageal reflux compared to the control and placebo" *(Mosaffa-Jahrom et al, 2016)*. So, it looks like the ancient Egyptians had something after all.

Similarly, Romans ate cakes stuffed with anise and other aromatic seeds to aid digestion. It was considered a "hot" seed by the Greeks and Romans, who recommended it as an aphrodisiac. Later, after the aphrodisiac had worked (I presume), nursing mothers were urged to ingest anise to improve the quality and quantity of their milk. As it turns out, anise does contain "estrogen-like chemicals" so there may be some truth in the traditional use as an aphrodisiac. Because of anise's similarity to estrogen, those with hormone sensitive conditions should avoid use.

3. BLACKBERRY

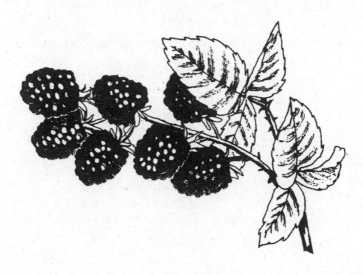

BOTANICAL NAME	*Rubus thunbergii*
PARTS USED	Leaves and bark

MEDICINAL REPUTATION	Soothing to all irritations and inflammations of the
	mucus membranes: nose, throat, stomach, and vagina, both orally in a tea and as a poultice.
	Relieves menstrual cramps.
	Prevents scurvy.
	Promotes virility and fertility.
	Highly recommended when treating cases of severe diarrhea (is there any other kind?).
REACTION	Nice, rich, leafy taste but without the muskiness found in raspberry leaf tea.
GRADE	B+

TRADITIONAL AND MODERN LORE

The fresh blackberry leaves rubbed on cuts and scratches were once considered to be highly beneficial. Of course, if you hadn't been out in the berry patch picking the blackberries, you wouldn't have gotten those cuts and scratches in the first place! It was considered useful as an antidote against the devil and assorted imps—large and small. However, this only works before October 11, the Old World's

Michaelmas Day, the day Lucifer was kicked out of heaven.

Blackberry tea was served to those in the throes of romantic entanglements: before, during, and after. By the way, blackberries make a lovely wine, rich and sweet. Just ask Mogen David or Manischewitz.

Research is being done at Brandeis University, Penn State University, the German equivalent of the FDA (Commission E), and the National Cancer Institute with intriguing results. Much of what the blackberry leaf tea has been used for in the past is now being substantiated.

The leaves are also reputed to be anti-inflammatory and have been used as poultices for sore muscles and inflammations. Taken orally, it does seem to relieve acute diarrhea. While blackberries do not lower the glycemic levels in your blood, as had been reported, their sugar content is so low that they do not raise your sugar levels. So far, no negative effects have been noted.

4. BLACK CURRANT

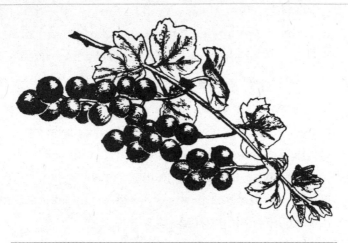

BOTANICAL NAME	*Ribes nigrum*
PARTS USED	Leaves
MEDICINAL REPUTATION	Deals predominantly with problems of the urinary tract: gravel, gout, water retention, inflammation.
	Soothes sore throats and colds.
	Controls stomach acid.
	Recommended as a superior thirst quencher in summers.
REACTION	Leafy, a little bland.
GRADE	B

TRADITIONAL AND MODERN LORE

Black currant was once considered to be an acceptable substitute for the Fountain of Youth. Since time out of mind, it has been said that those who drank black currant tea would remain youthful and the symptoms of old age would never manifest themselves.

This reputation would make sense given the medicinal properties of the black currant leaves/tea. Black currant leaves are high in Vitamin C and gamma-linolenic acid (GLA), which may improve the immune system. They are also a great source of anthocyanins, which are rich in antioxidants, and have antibacterial and antiviral properties.

We know that Vitamin C is good for us and our immune systems but the antioxidant/antiviral/antibacterial properties have led to some interesting and promising research in slowing cancer growth. Liver cancer cell growth was slowed when dosed with black currant extract, according to research by Northeastern Ohio Universities Colleges of Medicine and Pharmacy.

What they couldn't know, back in the day, was that the tea also reduces plaque buildup in the heart, spleen, kidneys, pancreas, and liver. That might explain the "Fountain of Youth" connection. It can also act as a blood thinner.

5. BORAGE

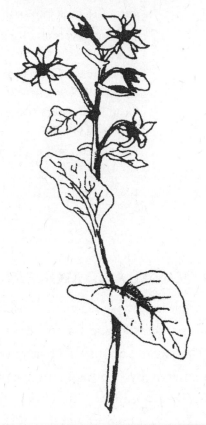

BOTANICAL NAME	*Borago officinalis*
PARTS USED	Leaves and flowers

MEDICINAL REPUTATION	High in potassium nitrate and calcium.
	Soothed inflamed eyes.
	Increases milk in nursing mothers.
	Reduces fevers and their accompanying coughs
	Used to rebuild strength after being cured of tuberculosis.
	Used for disorders of kidneys, liver, and bladder.
	Cheered up and gave "courage" to the consumer.
REACTION	Bland, cucumber-y flavor.
GRADE	B

TRADITIONAL AND MODERN LORE

Virtually every society—ancient and modern—knew and recommended borage for its "courage-giving" abilities. Then again, no one has particularly defined what was meant by "courage" or what situations demanded that courage. There may be a clue, however, in the fact that borage was once prescribed for the "lunatick person."

Borage tea is rich in GLA (*gamma linoleic acid* aka omega-6 fatty acid). This decreases inflammation in the body, and research is exploring possible applications for relieving asthma attacks by reduction of inflamed capillaries and veins in the lungs. It may also reduce the inflammation and pain of rheumatoid arthritis.

On the down side—there are also chemicals in borage that can damage liver cells and possibly even encourage some cancer cells.

CAUTION: This should be avoided by people who are pregnant and/or breastfeeding. Borage also contains small amounts of chemicals that may worsen liver toxicity.

6. CATNIP (CATMINT)

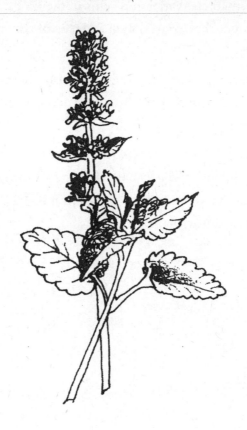

BOTANICAL NAME	*Nepeta cataria*
PARTS USED	Leaves

MEDICINAL REPUTATION	Calming to those prone to hysterics and/or nightmares.
	Eases menstrual cramps.
	"Cures" colds, smallpox, and scarlet fever.
	Used on colicky babies.
	Taken internally and externally to soothe pain of bruises and piles.
	A carminative—used to induce sweating without raising body temperature of fever victims.
	Extremely high in Vitamin C.
REACTION	Quite pleasant; a flavor of mint with perhaps a hint of cedar?
GRADE	B+

TRADITIONAL AND MODERN LORE

The 1735 *General Irish Herbal* is an early proponent of catnip tea and focuses on its value with tummy trouble: nausea, colic, cramps, and indigestion.

Early American pioneers used it as a poultice; gentle folk chewed it surreptitiously to bring on a little Dutch courage although catnip is actually calming, rather than stimulating, when ingested by humans. For further information about catnip's silliness value, consult your cats—if you can stop them from giggling long enough to talk to you! It's all about the chemical *nepetalactone* in the catnip that makes cats get the zoomies. It's strange then that catnip tea seems to have exactly the opposite effect on humans. Most (humans) find catnip tea very soothing and calming. Go figure.

Fun fact: nepetalactone drives off mosquitoes and cockroaches even more effectively than the leading profession bug repellent (DEET). The only problem is that it is a short-lived effect and needs to be reapplied every few hours.

7. CHAMOMILE (CAMOMILE)

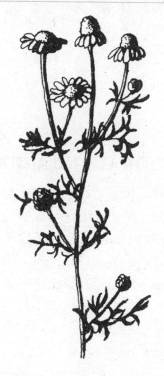

BOTANICAL NAME	*Matricaria chamomilla*
PARTS USED	Leaves and flowers

MEDICINAL REPUTATION	Eases severe menstrual cramps.
	A universal pain reliever.
	Generally enjoyed for its soothing, calming effect.
REACTION	A definite flavor of pineapple with a hint of chrysanthemums.
	Pleasing and refreshing.
GRADE	A

TRADITIONAL AND MODERN LORE

From earliest times, chamomile has been used for smelling, drinking, and burning purposes. Egyptians, Greeks, and Germans have associated the chamomile plant with gods—most likely for its healing properties which seemed heaven-sent. People loved it; fleas hated it. This was why it was common to scatter chamomile branches on the floors of castles—for cleanliness, a nice smell, and to keep the buggies away. Some scholars feel chamomile may have been the "lilies of the field" that Christ referred to since their abundance and growing season most closely fit the time, place, and context of the lesson.

Traditionally, it has been recommended for its sleep-inducing properties—which has been supported by modern research. Given this, it is recommended that you not "drink and drive" after more than one or two cups of the tea.

Once again, modern research is supporting the tradition that chamomile tea eases severe menstrual cramps. It is also being explored for its value in lowering or maintaining low blood sugar. It isn't a replacement for medication, but does seem to be a good supplement for helping to reduce complications of diabetes.

CAUTION: This is another tea that pregnant people should probably avoid.

⑧ COMFREY ROOT

(aka - Knitbone, Boneset, Healing Herb)

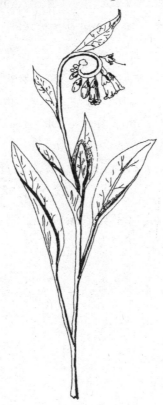

BOTANICAL NAME	*Symphytum officinale*
PARTS USED	Roots and leaves

MEDICINAL REPUTATION	Relieves inflamed and ulcerated wounds.
	Used both externally and internally to heal mouth and stomach ulcers.
	Eases severe pulmonary problems: asthma, bronchitis, tuberculosis.
	"Inhibited growth of malignant tumors."
	Used internally and externally to speed healing of fractured bones.
REACTION	A mild celery flavor, but most people found it pretty yucky. Since it is supposed to be so good for you, maybe it would be better in a soup stock?
GRADE	C-

TRADITIONAL AND MODERN LORE

The Crusaders were said to be impressed by the way the Turks were successfully treating their wounded with comfrey root concoctions. The Crusaders did likewise and were impressed enough with the results to bring the roots back with them to Europe.

Pilgrims, anticipating injuries while stealing an entire tectonic plate from its owners in order to design their New World, brought it to America with them. It was especially loved because it is both gentle and effective, making it useful for the very old and the very young alike.

HOWEVER! Comfrey also contains a chemical called *pyrrolizidine alkaloid* (PA). When you get through the Latin and Greek references, the bottom line is that comfrey can cause serious liver damage.

ALSO HOWEVER! That said, comfrey tea, when ingested, has been used for centuries to relieve ulcers, heavy menstrual flow, coughs, and angina. In a poultice, comfrey soothes aching muscles, varicose veins, gout and—oh yeah! Fractured bones.

CAUTION: Since there are serious safety concerns about the toxicity of this plant through skin absorption, pregnant people should absolutely avoid comfrey. It should be avoided by those with liver and kidney disease as well.

⑨ DANDELION

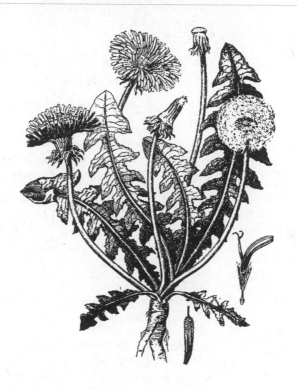

BOTANICAL NAME	*Taraxacum officinale*
PARTS USED	Leaves, flowers, roots

MEDICINAL REPUTATION	Very high in Vitamin C, iron, and potassium.
	Promotes general good health, especially of the heart, liver, and kidneys.
	Used as a diuretic in large doses.
	Used as a mild sedative.
	The strained tea is said to blanch freckles.
	The dried, roasted roots were ground to make a coffee which was used to provide relief from gout, jaundice, rheumatism, and hypochondria.
	Drinking the juice made by boiling the flowers was said to slow rapid heartbeat.
	The sap, placed on a wart and allowed to dry there, would cause warts to disappear.
REACTION	The young greens are great in salads. Slightly bitter/tangy in the way crisp greens and endive can be. The blossoms are delicious when dipped in tempura batter and fried. It's bitter but in the way some endive and some lettuces are.
GRADE	B+

TRADITIONAL AND MODERN LORE

The Greeks said that the dandelion sprang up in the tracks left by Apollo's sun chariot. Many myths were built up around the exploits of Theseus, famed Minotaur killer, involving the dandelion. It is said that Theseus ate the leaves and flowers of the dandelion for forty days before embarking on his exploits. It may also have been one of the five original bitter herbs used at the Passover Seder.

While there are no mentions of the dandelion specifically other than as a bitter herb in this traditional literature, eating dandelions after long periods of fasting and/or in high stress situations makes sense since they are loaded with vitamins A, C, and K. Vitamin K assists in blood clotting and slowing bleeding—which could be handy if you're taking on a Minotaur. In addition, dandelions contain lots of iron, calcium, magnesium, and potassium, all of which ensure muscle strength and agility.

Indigenous Americans chewed dandelion as a gum and pounded the blossoms into a paste to help heal broken bones. They believed that the dandelion was once a beautiful blonde maiden, beloved of the Wind. But before he could claim her, she became a white-haired old lady. In frustration, he blew all her hair away.

Europe had been imbibing dandelion tea for relief of liver and urinary problems. However, the French cautioned about drinking what they nicknamed *"pis en lit"* before bed: the French claimed it made the drinker pee the bed.

While there doesn't seem to be a great deal of genuine medical research done on the dandelion's supposed health-giving properties, virtually every culture from China to the Middle East to Europe all repeat the same information: it's good for you and it helps ease pee-pee problems.

CAUTION: Like everything else, overdoing eating the leaves should be avoided as they contain oxalates which have been implicated in kidney stones and gout. If you already have these conditions, maybe avoid dandelion greens.

⑩ EYEBRIGHT

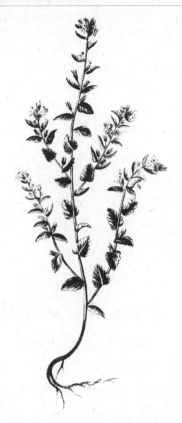

BOTANICAL NAME	*Euphrasia officinalis*
PARTS USED	Flowers, flowering stems, leaves

MEDICINAL REPUTATION	A cooled eyebright tea was used to bathe eyes suffering from conjunctivitis and other infections, irritation from hay fever, and dimness from old age.
	Relieves head cold distress.
	Comforts digestive disorders.
	Seems to alleviate pain of gallbladder
	attacks.
REACTION	Yucky
GRADE	D

TRADITIONAL AND MODERN LORE

There is very little information about eyebright to be found. What there is of it seems to center about its uses in nature: birds and snakes (in mythology) use eyebright for personal hygiene; birds used it to sharpen their eyesight; serpents recommended it to one another for restoring their eyesight after shedding their skins. Eyebright was grown in medieval monastery gardens and served in a conserve in order to brighten the eyesight of the monks.

Interestingly, modern research—what there is of it—shows that eyebright does have some chemicals (luteolin and quercetin) which (surprise!) have antihistamine properties which reduce inflammation and redness, especially in the eyes. A compound called *acubin* is included in eyebright's package. Some research has also indicated that it can ease oxidative damage and/or reduce scarring of heart tissue post-surgery.

11 FENNEL

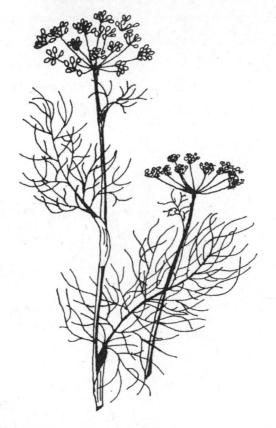

BOTANICAL NAME	*Foeniculum vulgare*
PARTS USED	Fronds, stems, seeds

MEDICINAL REPUTATION	Said to improve eyesight. It is the tummy's best friend: relieves nausea, constipation, may help manage weight, as well as stimulates the appetite. Eases the discomfort of fevers, cramps, and rheumatism. Oil of fennel was used locally on backaches and toothaches.
REACTION	Most people liked the licorice flavor; yummy
GRADE	B+

TRADITIONAL AND MODERN LORE

Puritans often chewed fennel seeds during their interminable church services to sweeten their breath. Fennel seeds sprinkled on doorways will prevent ghosts' unlawful entry. Sprigs of fennel were scattered throughout the house to ward off the evil eye. Outdoors, fennel was equally useful: the juice of fennel, when rubbed on cows' udders, prevented the milk from being bewitched. It was also used by snakes as an eyesight restorer after shedding their skins. If you like Italian food, you love fennel. No valid research has supported the idea that fennel helps *prevent* diabetes, however, since it is rich in fiber and low in the glycemic index, it does seem to ward off sugar spiking.

Because of its high amount of vitamin C, calcium, potassium, as well as an estrogen-like chemical and its antibacterial properties, it is a healthful drink. While there is no solid medical proof, these ingredients may help to explain its reputation for easing nausea, colicky babies, menstrual cramps, arthritis, and perhaps IBS.

CAUTION: Heavy use of fennel (as a tea, salad green, pizza topping, or spaghetti sauce/gravy) may lessen the effectiveness of birth control medications. Do not drink fennel while you are nursing your baby. The chemicals will be passed through to the baby through the breast milk. So don't do it!

12 FENUGREEK

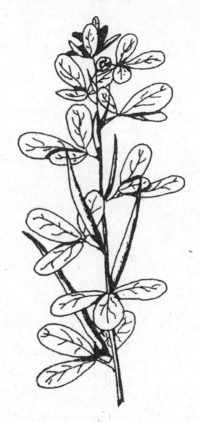

BOTANICAL NAME	*Trigonella foenum-graecum*
PARTS USED	Seeds and leaves

MEDICINAL REPUTATION	Was used for upset or gassy stomachs. Soothes sores in the mouth. A rich source of protein, fenugreek was reputed to cure baldness and promote a thick, glossy re-growth of hair. Fenugreek is now being researched as a possible source of ingredients used in the manufacture of oral contraceptives.
REACTION	A flavor like curry powder; few enjoyed it as a tea; again, better in a soup stock?
GRADE	C

TRADITIONAL AND MODERN LORE

The ancient Egyptians used fenugreek with a kind of a "kill or cure" approach. They seemed to believe that fenugreek could cure almost everything: generic body aches and pains, bronchitis, gout, swollen glands, and acne. Concubines used it to increase their beauty by plumping up their figures and thickening their hair. They also claimed it was not only an effective contraceptive but also helped pump up one's libido. If things didn't work out, fenugreek was used in preserving your mummy—and probably your daddy (Yes, I had to!). Fenugreek seeds were found in Tutankhamun's tomb—fat lot of good they did him. But that's another book.

Traditionally, cloisters in Europe grew fenugreek for all of its medicinal properties since the monks were often the more intelligent members of society and knew how to grow and apply medicinal herbs.

Those into alternative medical treatments feel that fenugreek can lower blood sugar spikes after a meal. Fenugreek is also said to relieve upset stomachs, heartburn, constipation, hardening of the arteries (and therefore atherosclerosis), gout, and baldness. There isn't much in the way of genuine medical proof of these claims, but they have stuck around for over 3000 years.

CAUTION: Fenugreek is not for those with hypoglycemia (low blood sugar) or blood clotting disorders. Also not good for pregnant people or those who are nursing.

13 GINGER

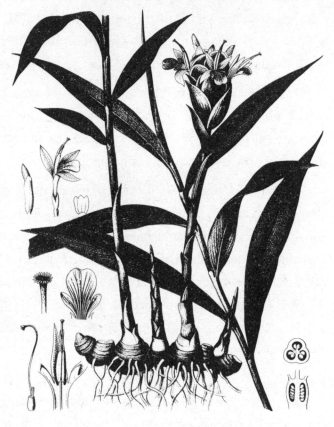

BOTANICAL NAME	*Zingiber officinale*
PARTS USED	Roots—fresh or dried and shredded

MEDICINAL REPUTATION	Resolves nausea and other upset stomach pains.
	Eases pain of arthritic knees.
REACTION	Yummy!
GRADE	A+

TRADITIONAL AND MODERN LORE

Ginger has been used medicinally for thousands of years. It was used by Austronesians (in Southeast Asia, Taiwan, Polynesia, etc.) to relieve nausea. In other physical healing rituals, ginger roots protected ships at sea. Roots of ginger were thrown overboard to calm and/or appease storms and the evil spirits associated with them

Today's medical research is substantiating the traditions ascribed to ginger's sick tummy helper. It has been especially helpful in relieving the nausea of patients in chemotherapy as well as those who are pregnant.

Exciting research is also showing that ginger seems to slow the advance of many cancers: liver, pancreatic, stomach, and colo-rectal.

CAUTION: Ginger is contraindicated if you are using blood thinners like Warfarin or even aspirin. Talk to your doctor. We are also getting mixed signals regarding ginger's use by people who are pregnant. Many doctors suggest avoiding it during pregnancy but at the same time suggesting ginger for relieving morning sickness. I can't help but wonder what medicines are prescribed in lieu of ginger and what their safety (profit??) levels are.

I'm paranoid. So sue me.

14 GINSENG

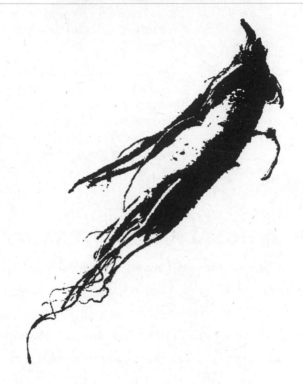

BOTANICAL NAME	*Panax quinquefolium*
PARTS USED	Roots only

MEDICINAL REPUTATION	Reputed to cure just about everything and anything that ails you. Best known for its reputation for restoring sexual virility in older folks.
REACTION	Everyone liked the spicy minty taste and many made it a point to buy their own supply. No one reported on their subsequent love lives, but there was a lot of giggling going on.
GRADE	A

TRADITIONAL AND MODERN LORE

This is one of the most mystical of all the herbs. It is renown in Chinese pharmacology as a panacea, particularly concerning, and especially focusing on, sexual dysfunction. Thus, the humanoid-shaped roots are literally worth their weight in gold.

Anthropologists and sociologists have reported vivid and complex dreams after ingesting bits of the root. Some Biblical scholars even claim that the bread supplied to Ezekiel by the ravens while he was meditating in the desert contained ginseng. They claim that this is what caused his hallucinations of flying ships and alien abduction.

The woods and hillsides of early (and present day) America were/are ransacked for the plant that grows wild there. There is still an active cultivation, exploitation, and exportation industry of the ginseng here because of the demand by asian and local herbalists. However, beware! If you choose to grow your own ginseng—and there is money to be made doing it—every article regarding the business advises that you never tell anyone what you are doing as there are really nasty ginseng rustlers out there. Seriously!

⑮ GOLDENSEAL

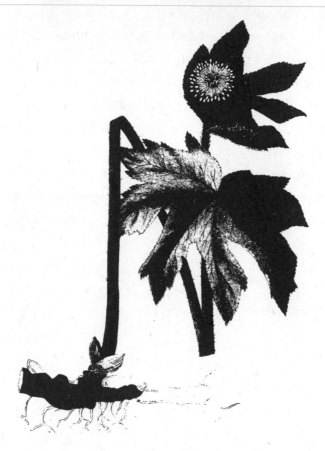

BOTANICAL NAME	*Hydrastis Canadensis*
PARTS USED	Rhizomes

MEDICINAL REPUTATION	Specialized in ailments of the mucous membrane of the nasal, gastro-intestinal, and genital-urinary tracts.
	Particularly recommended for vaginitis.
	Cools fevers, especially those associated with typhoid.
	Soothes the stomach.
	Can be a mild laxative.
REACTION	Bitter and somewhat unpleasant
GRADE	C

TRADITIONAL AND MODERN LORE

Goldenseal can be considered a stem to stern remedy: it has been used for everything from eye inflammation to hemorrhoids and pretty much everything in between—even the common cold. Indigenous Americans also used goldenseal as a dye and a highly effective insect repellent.

Goldenseal is included in many over-the-counter drugs for vaginitis, colds, UTI's, inflammations, upset stomachs, and hemorrhoids. This is because goldenseal contains rich deposits of berberine, hydrastine, and canadine, which are all antiinflammatory and antibacterial.

Widely prized for its effectiveness in dealing with the above ailments, foragers quickly denuded the landscape of golden seal. Its finicky growing habits make it difficult to propagate and cultivate. Because of this, you can make decent money growing goldenseal.

CAUTION: It has recently been associated with causing the mother to lose weight during pregnancy and may stimulate contractions and possibly endanger the fetus by inducing labor.

16 HIBISCUS

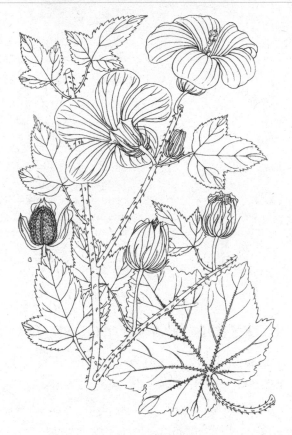

BOTANICAL NAME	*Hibiscus sabdariffa*
PARTS USED	Flowers, leaves, and occasionally roots

MEDICINAL REPUTATION	Worldwide reputation for lowering blood pressure and cholesterol.
	Aids in weight loss.
	High in Vitamin C and therefore an antioxidant.
	Used for liver disorders.
	Calms digestive disorders.
	Eases symptoms of cold and flu.
REACTION	Most people liked its floral, slightly tangy taste; it was familiar as it is used in many of the lemon-y tasting herbal tea combinations.
GRADE	B+

TRADITIONAL AND MODERN LORE

I challenge you to find a commercially packaged herbal tea mix that *doesn't* contain hibiscus flowers. For that matter, try to find a yard in Florida that isn't sporting hibiscus plants flowering away.

There doesn't seem to be much history attached to the hibiscus despite its popularity from China to the South Pacific to Florida. Some people in North Africa used it in a tea to induce a cooling sweat.

Research does support that hibiscus tea can help lower blood pressure, but it can be tricky for those who already have lower blood pressure issues. Fatigue, dizziness, and headache can also accompany this as sort of a package deal. Hibiscus also contains anthocyanins, which are beneficial to a healthy heart.

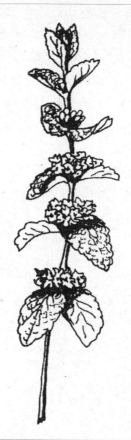

BOTANICAL NAME	*Marrubium vulgare*
PARTS USED	Flowering tips

MEDICINAL REPUTATION	Used for treating coughs and lung ailments.
	Stimulates poor heart function and promotes better circulation.
	Eases digestive problems.
	An antispasmodic.
	Indigenous Americans used it to increase urine and perspiration output.
REACTION	The strong, musky flavor took a little getting used to, but most people liked it. Many cough drops today include a base of horehound. There is also a hint of licorice.
GRADE	B+

TRADITIONAL AND MODERN LORE

The ancient Egyptians associated horehound with the most potent aspects of their most powerful gods. Their names for horehound were *seed of Horus* and *bull's blood (Apis)*. Greeks used it to counteract the poisons from the bite of a mad dog, snake, or too much booze. Ancient Romans used it to relieve respiratory problems. Today, some scholars believe horehound was another of the five bitter herbs used at the Passover Seder.

During the Middle Ages, horehound was also cultivated in monastery gardens for its medicinal properties. Horehound tea reduces inflammation in the circulatory system as well as in alveoli in the lungs, thus it can be soothing to asthmatics. The reduction in inflammation can also reduce heart attacks and/or their severity. This seems to extend to belly cramps and menstrual cramps. Some research indicates that horehound helps to lower LDL (bad cholesterol).

18 HYSSOP

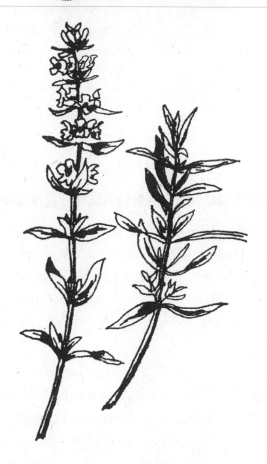

| BOTANICAL NAME | *Hyssopus officinalis* |
| PARTS USED | Tips of the young leaves |

MEDICINAL REPUTATION	Mildly stimulating.
	"Cleanses" blood and internal organs.
	Regulates blood pressure.
	Eases discomfort of respiratory complaints.
	Prevents sweating.
REACTION	Pleasant; faintly pine-y
GRADE	B+

TRADITIONAL AND MODERN LORE

Hyssop winds its way through the Bible as being a cleansing agent. The Temple was swept with hyssop branches for purification, as were places where the dead had lain. Houses preparing for holidays of renewal and rejoicing were swept and strewn with hyssop.

In Exodus, God orders the Jewish people to take branches of hyssop, dip them in the blood of the lamb that had been slaughtered for dinner the night of the first Passover in Egypt. They were to take the hyssop branches and smear their doorways with drops of the blood. That way the Angel of Death would know which houses to pass over.

Although there is still some confusion about exactly which plant went by the name of "hyssop," it is thought that it was the reed supporting the sponge soaked in sour wine which was lifted up to Christ on the Cross.

Traditionally, hyssop was used to cure lepers. The "recipe" also included some cedar wood, some scarlet wool, and a live bird (I have no idea!). However, it can be used as a poultice for bruises and boo boos. It also soothes irritations in the nose, throat, and lungs.

Hyssop has also figured prominently in some Gregorian chants and Plainsong in the Mass. Worshippers were/are sprinkled with hyssops dipped in holy water when leaving church after Mass. Perhaps that is why it was also reputed to ward off the evil eye.

CAUTION: Any form of hyssop taken internally or externally can cause serious problems for pregnant people and/or the fetus. Hyssop should be avoided if you are pregnant. Even more caution should be exercised by those prone to seizures, especially children, as hyssop may increase the frequency and intensity of the attacks.

⟨19⟩ LAVENDER

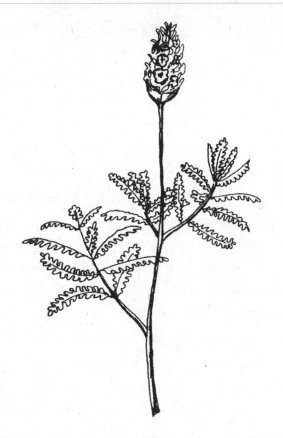

BOTANICAL NAME	*Lavandula angustifolia*
PARTS USED	Flowers and leaves

MEDICINAL REPUTATION	Calms nervousness, trembling, and hysteria
	Soothes hoarse and/or sore throats. Relieves migraines and sleeplessness.
	Aided in digestion as an antispasmodic.
	Prevents sunstroke.
	Cured "passion of the heart."
	Warded off the Black Plague.
REACTION	Very exotic; like drinking perfume.
GRADE	B

TRADITIONAL AND MODERN LORE

Like hyssop, lavender (from the Latin *lavare*—to wash) appears repeatedly in the Bible. On their way out of the Garden of Eden, Adam and Eve were said to have grabbed a few plants. Probably because it smells so good, but also they may have sensed its many useful properties: as an antibacterial, sanitizer, and its ability to ward off the evil eye.

When Mary Magdalene washed Jesus' feet, it is believed that she used lavender and/or spikenard. The two are used interchangeably, but they are not really related horticulturally.

The dried blossoms were the original smelling salts. The Romans perfumed their baths with it (so do we). Queen Elizabeth I ate it as a conserve while her subjects wore sprigs of lavender in their caps to ward off colds, mental disorders, and possibly plague and tuberculosis. Lavender may be what the song, "Ring around a rosie, pocket full of posies," is referring to. "Ring around a rosie" refers to the appearance of a circular red ring on the inflamed skin of someone infected with the Plague. "Pocket full of posies" refers to the tradition of keeping sprigs of lavender in their pockets to ward off Plague infection.

Modern research has shown that indeed, lavender has a highly toxic effect on such bacilli as diphtheria, typhoid, tuberculosis (Koch's bacillus), and pneumonia. Lately there have been claims that children on the autism spectrum find the fragrance especially soothing.

⓴ LEMON VERBENA

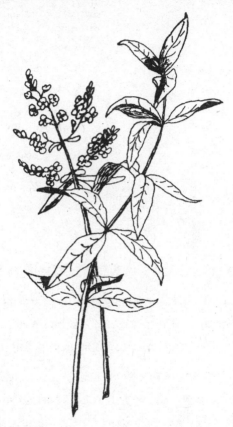

BOTANICAL NAME	*Lippia citriodora*
PARTS USED	Leaves

MEDICINAL REPUTATION	Once used as an antidote to snakebite.
	Prescribed for ulcers, dropsy (edema or water retention), gout, and jaundice.
	Relieves heartburn.
	An antispasmodic.
	Calms asthmatic and/or nervous coughs.
REACTION	Delicious! Has a lemony, leafy flavor. Best served as iced tea.
GRADE	A+

TRADITIONAL AND MODERN LORE

Lemon verbena flowers were said to have been born from the tears of Juno, queen of the Greek pantheon, when one of her favorite mortals was killed.

Dioscorides (40-90 AD) recommended lemon verbena as a poultice or tea to treat attacks by harvest spiders, dogs, and/or scorpions. Charlemagne (742-814 AD) used it and had it planted all over his gardens as he seemed to believe it would keep him young. He lived to be over seventy, so . . .

Nicholas Culpeper, the famous herbalist from the 1600's, reinforced Charlemagne's belief and said that lemon verbena tea made the heart merry. As did the scientist Paracelsus.

Plucked from their native volcanic slopes of South America, the verbenas were transported back to Spain by the conquistadores. Lemon verbena is also a favorite for warding off evil spirits amongst modern day druids.

There is some research—but nothing conclusive yet—concerning lemon verbena's use in treating multiple sclerosis. And while it is soothing and can help you get a restful night's sleep, don't use it if you are already using sleep medication. Does the word "overdose" mean anything to you?

㉑ LINDEN FLOWER

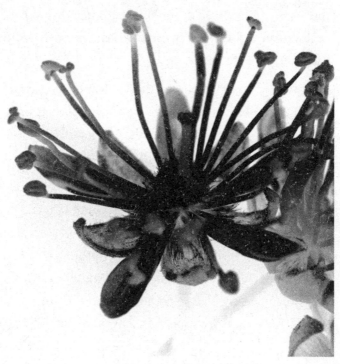

BOTANICAL NAME	*Tilia x europaea*
PARTS USED	Flowers, flowering tips

MEDICINAL REPUTATION	Helps to lower high blood pressure and reduce arteriosclerosis.
	Good for colds, sore throats, and hoarseness.
	Promotes sweating to help reduce fever.
	Used by sufferers of vertigo, edema, migraine, epilepsy, and paralysis.
	Halts diarrhea.
	An antispasmodic.
REACTION	A combination of flowers with a hint of cardboard; it might be better when brewed from fresh ingredients.
GRADE	B+

TRADITIONAL AND MODERN LORE

Women in primitive societies used the Linden groves for their rituals while the menfolk were whooping it up in the oak groves. The linden symbolized maternal love to the Greeks, and Catholic tradition uses the linden's heart-shaped leaf to represent the sacred heart of Jesus. In both Germany and the East, trials were often held under the linden's branches. It was believed that the leaves induced a sense of justice and conciliation to all parties involved. Linden has been thought to be the tree whose branches caught up the hair of King David's treacherous son, Absalom, holding him until he was executed.

Used in conjunction with spider webs (beats me), linden would ward off the Plague. Because of its beauty, fragrance, and medicinal properties, the linden tree was used to line city streets by orders of the kings. France planted 60,000 linden trees throughout Paris after the end of the French Revolution. You will still see many streets in Europe lined with these (extremely photogenic) trees. Possibly due to this beauty, linden groves are supposed to be the most fortuitous places for love making. (I'm not sure what they mean by "fortuitous.")

The leaves, bark, and especially the flowers should be included when making the mixture for brewing.

22 NETTLE

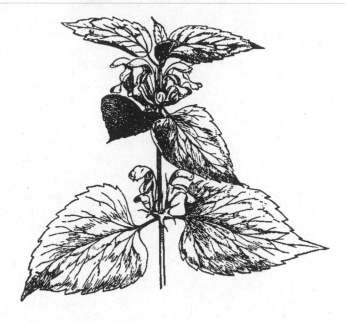

BOTANICAL NAME	*Urtica dioica*
PARTS USED	Leaves, including stingers

MEDICINAL REPUTATION	High in Vitamins A and C.
	Used to help lose weight.
	Hot tea gives luster to the hair and eyes.
	Cold tea cures dandruff.
	When brewed as a beer, said to relieve pain of gout.
	Seeds, bruised in white wine, supposedly helps expel bladder stones.
	Nettles were rubbed on rheumatic joints, serving as a counter-irritant to the pain (of course, so will hitting yourself on the toes with a hammer).
REACTION	Delicious! Can easily be substituted for "regular" tea.
GRADE	A+

TRADITIONAL AND MODERN LORE

Norse gods were fond of the nettle. Loki, the Norse trickster god, used a magic fishing net made of nettles. His plan was to disguise himself as a fish and avoid Thor's anger. But Thor figured out how to make a net like Loki's and used it to catch him, then tied him to a rock and tortured him for the rest of time.

The nettle also appears in European fairy tales as a food source (not unlike spinach when the young, stinger-less leaves are boiled). Magical beings also turned it into a lovely thread for making gowns and as a substitute for flaxen thread. When the Romans invaded chilly Britain, they rubbed nettles all over their naked bodies and the resultant stinging kept them warm all day. (I'll stick to my electric blanket and my cuddly dachshund).

Victor Hugo refers to nettles in *Les Misérables* as being used by peasants as a food source for themselves and their cattle. It was also useful as a dye and medicine. These uses were revived during World War I by the Germans: the high protein content does actually make it an excellent cattle feed. It also turns out that a very acceptable linen-like fiber can indeed be made from nettles.

Science is also taking a new look at the nettle as a way to alleviate the pain of osteoarthritis. Further studies on rats are suggesting that the nettle may also help control sugar imbalances for diabetics and even control blood pressure.

㉓ PAPAYA

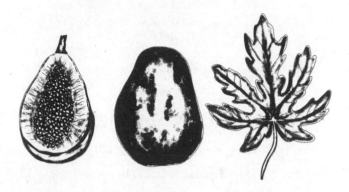

BOTANICAL NAME	*Carica papaya* (*aka* paw-paw)
PARTS USED	Leaves
MEDICINAL REPUTATION	Derivatives of papaya used in reducing swellings of inflammation or bruising.
	Serves as a catalytic agent in the manufacture of some antibiotics.
	Cleanses wounds.
	Aids digestion.
	Used in India to cure warts, freckles, and unsightly skin blemishes.
	Used to expel intestinal worms.

REACTION	Those worms are right about wanting to get away from this stuff! I wouldn't recommend it to a vulture. Some sites suggest adding salt to the tea. UGH!
GRADE	Z-

TRADITIONAL AND MODERN LORE

You might have heard that the villains in many ailments are called *free radicals*. These are atoms who are incomplete: they need another electron. So they roam through the body grabbing electrons from any atom they can which messes up the original atom so that it can't do its normal job. The results of this can cause cancer, various forms of heart disease, and possibly Alzheimer's.

BUT ingesting foods that are high in antioxidants will block the evil free radicals. Fresh papaya is loaded with antioxidants. This may be why some research is indicating that papaya leaf tea helps to block cancer cell growth. It may also be beneficial to people with gluten allergies, as the tea helps break down difficult to digest gluten molecules.

24 PARSLEY

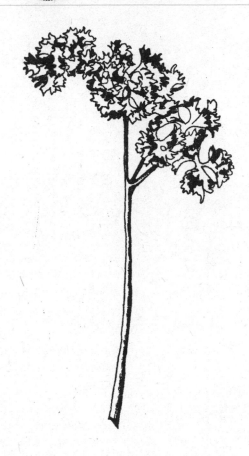

BOTANICAL NAME	*Petroselinum crispum*
PARTS USED	Leaves and stems

MEDICINAL REPUTATION	Rich in Vitamin C, iron, folate, iodine.
	An antiinflammatory and antioxidant.
	Said to be effective in treatment of lung, prostate, and colon cancers.
	Used for kidney stones.
	May lower blood pressure.
	Eases menstrual cramps and PMS.
	Used to cure acne.
	A mild diuretic.
	Relieves painful urinary and prostate inflammations.
	Used for curing liver ailments.
	A source for *cepyol*, which is used to treat malaria victims.
REACTION	No doubt about it, it's parsley alright! A medicinal, but with a good-for-you kind of bitterness.
GRADE	B

TRADITIONAL AND MODERN LORE

Parsley was said to have sprung up from the blood of Archemorus while he was being eaten by snakes. Thus, parsley has been traditionally associated with death and oblivion.

The Greeks crowned their champions and tombs with the wreaths of parsley (I don't quite get the connection, myself). Parsley was also sacred to Persephone, erstwhile wife of Hades, possibly because parsley roots are reputed to grow down as deep as Hell itself.

Perhaps, because of this, it was also said to figure prominently in witches' rites. Certainly, parsley has a magical effect on alleviating garlic breath.

In England, the term "Welsh parsley" was a euphemism for the hangman's noose. It was said that if parsley appeared in your garden, someone in the house would die within the year.

Several cultures associated consuming parley with inducing epileptic seizures, but I couldn't find any medical support for this.

CAUTION: If you are pregnant, parsley tea should not be drunk in any quantity as it can be harmful to the baby.

25 PEPPERMINT

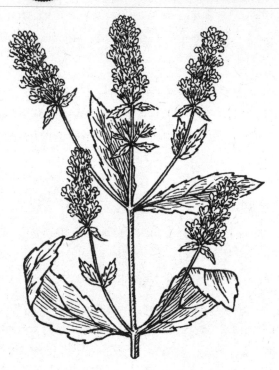

BOTANICAL NAME	Mentha x Piperita (For botany buffs, peppermint is a hybrid plant: a cross between spearmint and watermint.)
PARTS USED	Leaves

MEDICINAL REPUTATION	Relieves many stomach disorders: nausea, diarrhea, cramps, spasms.
	Soothes headaches from simple ones to migraines to hangovers.
	Said to have antiseptic and disinfectant properties.
	Rumored to have cured some cases of gangrene.
REACTION	After all the experimenting, this one was blessedly familiar—and delicious.
GRADE	A+

TRADITIONAL AND MODERN LORE

Greek mythology claims that Persephone, wife of Hades, got jealous of the nymph, Minthe. Never cross a jealous wife. She turned Minthe into a low-lying plant so that everyone would stomp on her.

The Bible refers to peppermint as an acceptable form of tithe payment. It has been scattered in temples, palaces, and humbler homes for its fragrance and possible disinfectant properties. Traditionally, cloth saturated in peppermint oil and/or tea was used to relieve tension headaches, sinus headaches, and even migraines. Travelers chewed it to prevent (or deal with) motion sickness, and empirical evidence tells us that peppermint does soothe upset tummies, nausea, vomiting, and can relieve gas. Medical research substantiates that peppermint does ease the pain and other symptoms of Irritable Bowel Syndrome (IBS). Used externally, peppermint tea takes the sting out of being stung.

26 RASPBERRY

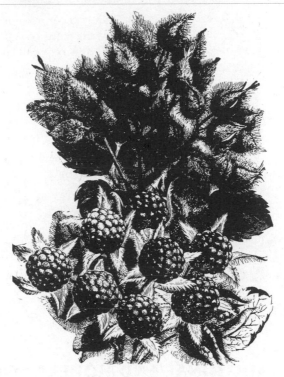

BOTANICAL NAME	*Rubus idaeus*
PARTS USED	Leaves

MEDICINAL REPUTATION	Relieves menstrual cramps, nausea, diarrhea, and vomiting.
	Widely recommended to ease the pains of difficult and/or prolonged labor.
	Cools fevers by inducing sweating.
	Prevents gray hair.
	"Fastens" teeth.
	Cures "eyes which hang out."
	Also used as an aphrodisiac.
REACTION	Exotic; a leafy taste with (surprise!) a strong flavor of unsweetened raspberries.
GRADE	B+

TRADITIONAL AND MODERN LORE

According to Greek mythology, raspberries were originally white. However, when the infant Jupiter had a crying spell, his babysitter, the nymph Ida, picked some of the luscious berries to calm him down. But the thorns pricked her fingers causing them to bleed and turned the berries red from then on.

Germans in the Middle Ages felt a raspberry cane tied to a difficult horse would tame him by warding off evil spirits. Filipinos also tied raspberry canes to their front doors to ward off evil spirits. The plant was also used by Indigenous Americans as a treatment for indigestion or gastrointestinal issues. HOWEVER! Too much of it can have exactly the opposite effect. One or two cups a day is the limit.

Raspberry leaf tea is now being researched as a source of treatment for schistosomiasis (an often fatal, snail-transmitted disease found in rivers). While modern medicine is still ambivalent about raspberry leaf tea easing the contractions during labor, over the centuries, many women have said it helps ease labor pains. In addition, because of its high potassium content, raspberry leaf tea can help keep blood pressure down. This may explain the reference to "eyes which hang out," as high blood pressure may put pressure on the eyeballs themselves.

27 RED CLOVER

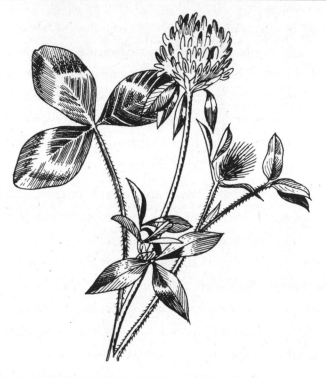

BOTANICAL NAME	*Trifolium pratense*
PARTS USED	Flowers

MEDICINAL REPUTATION	High vitamin C content. Used to "tone up the organs."
	Taken to cure colds.
	Reputed to cure insanity.
	Has been a source of dicumarol, an anticoagulant used on patients prone to blood clots.
REACTION	Pleasant, but just about what you would expect a tea from dried grass would taste like.
GRADE	B

TRADITIONAL AND MODERN LORE

St. Patrick used the clover to illustrate God's Plan. Clover plants have either three leaves (representing each member of the Trinity) or four leaves (representing how all three members of the Trinity are a whole), therefore, it is considered to have mystical properties. Legend says that clover was part of the bedding for the Christ Child's manger. It has been used to ward off the attentions of devils (and maybe of the IRS?).

Both in the Old World and the New, clover has been used for lawns, as a crop, and, when the manure ran out, a nitrogen-rich source of organic fertilizer. Of course, and possibly most importantly, bees love clover. Reminder—to paraphrase Albert Einstein's observation—"If the bees die out, Man has about four years left."

It is touted as relieving everything from the pain of menopause, asthma, heart issues, and now even cancer. While research is underway, there is no real medical consensus supporting these claims. It is, however, known that red clover should be avoided by those with hormone-sensitive conditions.

28 ROSE HIPS

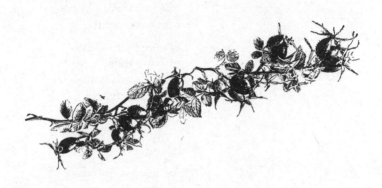

BOTANICAL NAME	*Rosa: rugosa, gallica, damascene, etc.* There are more than 30,000 varieties of roses out there with more coming every day!
PARTS USED	Rose hips (that red bulb left over at the top of the stem when the petals drop off), occasionally petals are included in salads.

MEDICINAL REPUTATION	Nearly 60 times higher in Vitamin C than in an equal weight of oranges—which is why nearly every herbal tea mix out there contains rose hips/petals.
	Has been used for treating those with tuberculosis and other lung disorders.
	Used to treat many (unspecified) mental disorders.
	Another "cure" for hydrophobia.
REACTION	Tangy! Fruity, with a hint of roses in the aftertaste. Delicious!
GRADE	A+

TRADITIONAL AND MODERN LORE

The part that roses have played in mythology, religion, and history is too extensive to go into any real depth here, but here are a couple of interesting ones: After the god Uranus (*aka* Ouranos) invented the heavens and earth, he turned on his rebellious son, Chronos, and imprisoned him. Chronos got even but cutting off his father's genitals and throwing them in the sea. There, Uranus' blood was transformed into roses. Another fun fact is that when the god Eros got stung by a bee while sniffing a rose, he went crying to his mommy, Aphrodite. His overprotective mommy soothed him by giving him a bow and arrows. He immediately shot the offending rose bush full of arrows—and that's why roses have thorns.

One particularly beautiful Christian legend mentions that those who first ventured into the tomb of the Virgin Mary found only heaps of fragrant lilies and roses. "Witches" throughout Europe used rose hips in their "magic" potions to cure scurvy, colds, and other things that are now treated with Vitamin C.

Indigenous Americans were doing the same thing in the other hemisphere—using rose tea to cure various ailments. Historically, there were many traditional concoctions prescribed for the comforting of the "melancholic." Modern research has in fact isolated a property in rose fragrance which does have an antidepressant effect. Lab animal research on the chemical compounds found in roses has concluded that some of its chemicals do indeed have something of a soporific ability.

29 ROSEMARY

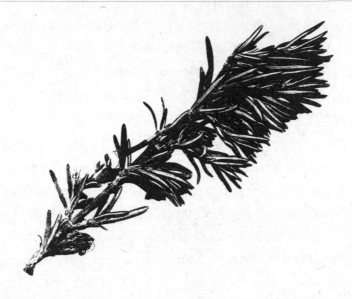

BOTANICAL NAME	*Rosmarinus officinalis*
PARTS USED	Leaves, flowering tips

MEDICINAL REPUTATION	Stimulates the brain— especially the memory.
	Relieves nervous tension.
	Frequently recommended for migraine headaches.
	Aids digestion by relieving gas and bloat.
	Increased bile flow.
	Relieves "female complaints."
	A mild diuretic.
	Sweetens breath.
	Rosemary oil was used to ease stiffness of rheumatic joints.
REACTION	Pine-y; very fragrant and pleasantly so.
GRADE	B+

TRADITIONAL AND MODERN LORE

Rosemary was grown in King Solomon's gardens as a source of incense. It was said to help ward off evil spirits and/or bad dreams. The flowers themselves are said to have derived their heavenly blue color from when the Holy Mother spread Her blue cloak as a blanket on a bed of rosemary on the weary flight to Egypt. Because of its devotion to the Holy Family, rosemary is said to refuse to live longer than thirty-three years: Christ's age when He was Crucified; nor will the plant exceed His height.

It was also said that inhaling its perfume will enhance your beauty and prolong your life. Donna Izabella of Hungary distilled a liqueur from rosemary which she faithfully drank every day. It must have worked because the King of Poland fell instantly in love with her and proposed marriage on the spot. And Donna Izabella was 72 years old and wracked with gout! And rich.

Today, research is beginning to support the tradition of rosemary tea easing menstrual cramps. Again, its high Vitamin C (an antioxidant) makes it useful for relieving colds and possibly slowing cancer. It's also a great way to help you get to sleep!

30 SAINT JOHN'S WORT

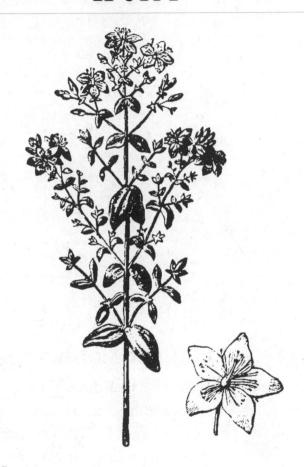

BOTANICAL NAME	*Hypericum perforatum*
PARTS USED	The whole plant, especially the flowers
MEDICINAL REPUTATION	Used for the last 2000 years as an antidepressant.
	Relieves insomnia and SAD (Seasonal Affect Disorder).
	Reduces wounds, cold sores, infections, and eczema.
	Possibly a blood thinner.
	Relieves symptoms of menopause.
	Reduces swelling of hemorrhoids.
	May also help to lower blood pressure.
REACTION	"Meh. It's okay," was the general consensus.
GRADE	B

TRADITIONAL AND MODERN LORE

St. John's wort may have been given its name from the color of the juice the blossoms exude when squeezed between the fingers: the color of the blood of the martyred saint, St. John. It was burned in doorways or other rooms to ward off or drive away evil spirits.

Traditionally, St. John's wort has been used as an antidepressant, anxiety reliever, and to generally soothe the nervous system. Those going through the process of giving up cigarettes, drugs, liquor, etc. find using St. John's helpful.

Recent research indicates that Saint John's wort, used in high doses, may help to lessen the effects of AIDS, hepatitis, and other viruses. The problem is that these dosages are so high that there can be serious negative effects as well. Research continues . . .

CAUTION: May adversely affect users of prescribed antidepressants, digoxin, cancer medications, blood thinners, and cyclosporine. It can also cause extreme sensitivity to sunlight and ultraviolet light. Severe sunburns can occur. It should also be avoided by those who are pregnant or breastfeeding.

㉛ SPEARMINT

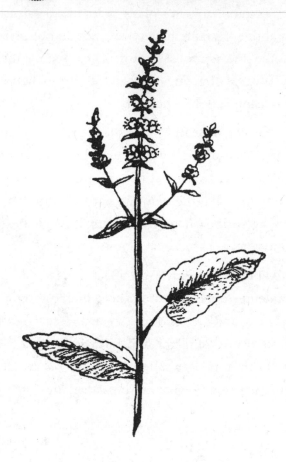

BOTANICAL NAME	*Mentha spicata*

PARTS USED	Leaves and stems
MEDICINAL REPUTATION	Cleanses and sweetens breath.
	Stimulates sexual ability.
	Once thought to prevent conception when ingested by either party involved.
	If not, then it was drunk mixed with wine to ease the pangs of childbirth.
REACTION	Exactly what we expected; refreshing.
GRADE	A

TRADITIONAL AND MODERN LORE

Ancient Hebrews scattered spearmint leaves and stems throughout the Temple to perfume the halls, and spearmint is used as one of the five bitter herbs at the Passover Seder. The Romans used it for "personal daintiness" as a deodorant and breath sweetener.

Today, experiments on cattle found that spearmint may lower blood pressure by reducing the severity of the contractions in blood vessels. They aren't sure if this applies to people. Yet.

Since spearmint does contain antitoxins, it is being looked at as an ally against heart disease and even cancer. And medical as well as empirical evidence still substantiates that it is useful for nausea and other tummy upsets.

32 TANSY

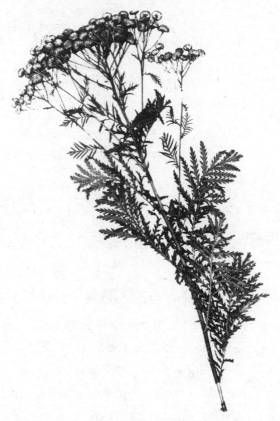

BOTANICAL NAME	*Tanacetum vulgare*
PARTS USED	Leaves and flowering tips

MEDICINAL REPUTATION	Thought to expel intestinal worms.
	Stimulates digestion.
	Helps to ease high blood pressure, heart problems, blood disorders.
	Alleviates menstrual cramps, nausea, and morning sickness.
	May ease pain of rheumatism (not necessarily the same thing as rheumatoid arthritis) and arthritis.
REACTION	Intriguingly bitter
GRADE	B

TRADITIONAL AND MODERN LORE

The early Greeks and Romans used tansy as a symbol of immortality. In fact, its name is derived from the Greek for "immortal." But it is not clear if they meant that taking tansy tea made you immortal or it preserved your remains for eternity.

Early settlers in New England would pack a coffin with it to preserve the body. Tansy pudding was served at the end of the forty days' fast to signal that Lent was over. The British herbalist Culpeper recommended tansy to women who desired children. Apparently, it was almost as effective as a husband, but I haven't figured out in just what capacity. Italians would hand a spring of tansy to an enemy as an insult and an open declaration of war.

When making your tea, remember that whatever part of the plant grows above the ground is safe; the roots can be poisonous. Keep in mind that the leaves of rhubarb (which contain oxalic acid) and potatoes (which contain deadly nightshade) are also dangerous, which is why you never see their leaves in the grocery store.

CAUTION: Moderation is the key to tansy. Ingesting large amounts of it has a reputation for reversing all of its positive effects! It can be fatal in large doses.

33 (WILD) STRAWBERRY

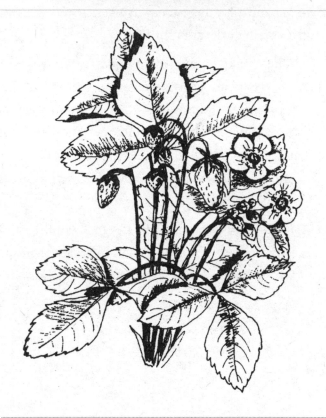

BOTANICAL NAME	*Fragaria vesca*
PARTS USED	Leaves

MEDICINAL REPUTATION	Thought to clean out the cleansing organs: liver, spleen, bladder, kidneys.
	High in iron and Vitamin C.
	Associated with lowering high blood pressure.
	Used for anemia.
	"Cured" gout.
	Relieves chronic diarrhea.
	A good gargle for sore throats.
	Reduces inflammation of wounds.
	Promotes virility and fertility.
REACTION	WOW! Super terrific! After this, "regular" tea is just plain boring.
GRADE	A+++++

TRADITIONAL AND MODERN LORE

In the spirit of ecumenism, the strawberry has been the personal favorite of higher beings from Venus to the Norse goddess Freja (from whom we got the word "Friday") to the Virgin Mary. In all cases, the strawberry is linked with love—causing it, maintaining it, enriching it.

The Chinese drank strawberry leaf tea to increase and improve longevity. Bavarian cattle had bags of strawberry fastened to their horns to increase and enrich their milk.

Other than the above references, strangely enough, there is very little mythology or traditional information about the strawberry. Maybe because it is just so good—between berries and tea leaves— there was no need to build it up.

CAUTION: If making your own tea, leaves MUST be thoroughly and completely dry. Moldy leaves can make you really, really sick!

34 VERVAIN

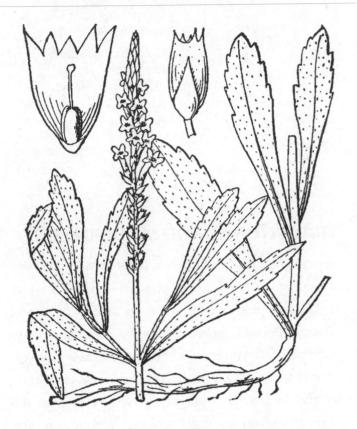

BOTANICAL NAME	*Verbena officinalis*
PARTS USED	Leaves and flowering tips

MEDICINAL REPUTATION	Another organ cleanser: tones up the liver, spleen, bladder, kidneys, etc.
	Calms migraines and nervous conditions.
	Eases various stomach disorders: cramps, diarrhea, flatulence.
	Relieves menstrual cramps.
REACTION	Bland and faintly bitter
GRADE	B-

TRADITIONAL AND MODERN LORE

Vervain has always been used for magic and was considered to be very powerful when casting spells. Its predominant use is in love potions and charms. Persians believed that by rubbing vervain on your body, you would become irresistible. It was eaten, drunk, touched, or rubbed onto your body to grant one's heart's desire. The Greeks took the opposite position—that rubbing vervain on you would drive away your enemies. It was said that vervain was used to wash the Body of Christ when He was being prepared for burial. Druids had a *quid pro quo* system: if you picked vervain, you had to replace it with a piece of honeycomb. They also believed that vervain was good for the kidneys. The Celtic name for vervain means "drives (kidney) stones away."

Ancient German hunters rubbed vervain on their weapons to ward off curses and to bring them luck in the hunt. With a similar philosophy of using the herb to protect against evil, parents would make their children wear vervain charms to ensure the child's good behavior and personality.

Today, modern research continues to support historical uses of vervain. There is one caveat however, do not expect vervain to *cure* these symptoms, but they may alleviate things. *Cornin,* a chemical found in glycoside, which is an element found in vervain, is known for clearing pathways to the heart and is considered to protect the heart. It has been found to be especially effective for healing myocardial ischemia.

Not unsurprisingly, vervain's chemicals also soothe intestinal linings as an anti-inflammatory.

Animal research has indicated that vervain has slowed cancerous growths. Vervain is high in the chemical *citral* which is a proven cancer inhibitor. It also contains flavonoids (back to the antioxidants), glycosides (they make sugar available to the body), and triterpenoids (also help maintain sugar levels and an antioxidant). It can be a diuretic and helpful in liver and kidney diseases. Some use it to treat depression.

CAUTION PREGNANT PEOPLE: Vervain had a reputation for increasing breastmilk production but modern research disputes this. In large doses, vervain may cause harm to the baby. Avoid it.

35 VIOLET

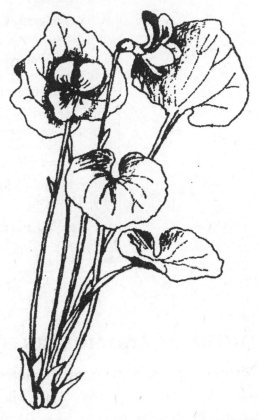

BOTANICAL NAME	Viola odorata
PARTS USED	Leaves and flowers

MEDICINAL REPUTATION	Used in Europe for relief of pulmonary problems: bronchitis, asthma, tuberculosis.
	Relieves migraines and other headaches.
	Given to children to "cure" them of epilepsy and/or convulsions.
	Used to help dissolve "mouth cancers" (probably what we call canker sores today).
	Taken in normal doses, is a *mild* laxative.
REACTION	Very pleasant and tea-y, but no one noticed any taste of violets.
GRADE	B+

TRADITIONAL AND MODERN LORE

The Violet is reputed to have sprung up from the blood of the Trojan War hero, Ajax, who killed himself in a fit of pique because he felt that *he* had been the MVP of the Trojan War. Therefore, he deserved to be given the magical armor of the now late Achilles. Instead, the armor was awarded to Odysseus.

Jupiter fed violet blossoms as a consolation to Princess Io after Juno changed the poor girl into a heifer as punishment for having had an affair with Jupiter. In Christian theology, ever since the Crucifixion, the violet always looks down, shunning the face of Man.

Elizabethan lovers used violets in a variety of charms to capture a lover and Napoleon took the plant as his personal emblem and presented large bouquets of it to Josephine on each of their wedding anniversaries. Sugared violets have long been a favorite European confection and breath sweetener.

Violet tea acts as a double whammy—as an anti-inflammatory, it reduces blood pressure, and also acts as a diuretic. It is soothing to the mucous membranes, thus reducing hoarseness, coughs, cold symptoms, and reducing the accompanying fever.

Research is showing that the leaves (and their high antioxidant value) may help reduce cancerous tumors.

CAUTION: Don't drink violet tea in large quantities because to do so would reverse all of its good effects. (Of course, that applies to almost everything we eat or drink, no?)

36 YARROW

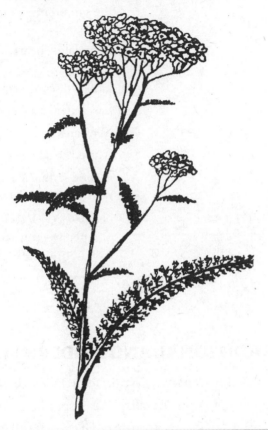

BOTANICAL NAME	*Achillea millefolium*
PARTS USED	Flowers and new leaves

MEDICINAL REPUTATION	Long considered to be a good overall tonic.
	Used to treat colds and the symptoms associated with colds.
	Stimulates "heart action."
	Soothing to stomach and kidney discomforts.
	Eases menstrual cramps.
	Alleviates gas.
	"Cured" baldness.
	A good styptic if you nick yourself when shaving.
REACTION	People either loved it or hated it—quite bitter with a strong flavor of cedar.
GRADE	B

TRADITIONAL AND MODERN LORE

Chiron the Centaur gave it to Achilles (hence the Latin designation "Achillae") as a specific prevention against war wounds. Chiron got it from the plants that grew in the rust on Achilles' shield and, from there, Achilles rubbed it on anyone who was wounded.

Apparently, Chiron forgot to advise Achilles to smear the juice of the yarrow on his heels.

Witches prescribed yarrow for conjuring up the image of one's beloved: sew a sprig of yarrow into a little piece of flannel, put it under your pillow, and fix it firmly in your mind that you expect to dream of your true love. Keeping yarrow about your person will guarantee that they will remain faithful and loving.

Science has backed up Chiron's advice: studies done on animals in Africa support the idea that yarrow may speed up the clotting and healing processes of wounds. Yarrow is also said to help regulate women's menstrual cycles and lower blood pressure. Yarrow has also been thought to help relieve anxiety and ease asthma attacks.

HOWEVER: If you are pregnant or planning to undergo surgery, it's best to avoid yarrow for the duration.

About the Author

Glenna McLean, M.S.Ed. began her writing career by editing and typing military R&D research project reports, including the flight manuals for the Apollo Projects. And the F-14 (See *Top Gun* for further clarification.) She spent the next 50 years teaching English in high school, college, and university, then ran her own state-accredited private school in Palm Beach for 15 years. She currently spends her time speaking, writing, editing, and cuddling and feeding animals.

Index

MORE HERBS FOR HEALTH

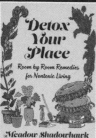
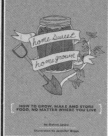
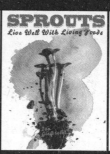
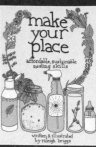

SUBSCRIBE!

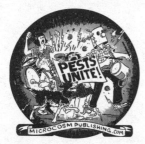

For as little as $15/month, you can support a small, independent publisher and get every book that we publish—delivered to your doorstep!

www.Microcosm.Pub/BFF

MORE NATURE FOR GETTING YOUR LIFE RIGHT

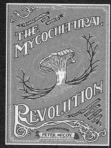
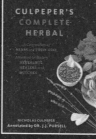
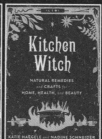
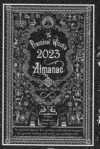